Paleo for Beginners

All about the Paleo Diet

How to Get Healthy & Lose Weight

By: Joanne Outram

PUBLISHERS NOTES

Disclaimer

This publication is intended to provide helpful and informative material. It is not intended to diagnose, treat, cure, or prevent any health problem or condition, nor is intended to replace the advice of a physician. No action should be taken solely on the contents of this book. Always consult your physician or qualified health-care professional on any matters regarding your health and before adopting any suggestions in this book or drawing inferences from it.

The author and publisher specifically disclaim all responsibility for any liability, loss or risk, personal or otherwise, which is incurred as a consequence, directly or indirectly, from the use or application of any contents of this book.

Any and all product names referenced within this book are the trademarks of their respective owners. None of these owners have sponsored, authorized, endorsed, or approved this book.

Always read all information provided by the manufacturers' product labels before using their products. The author and publisher are not responsible for claims made by manufacturers.

Trade Paperback Edition

Manufactured in the United States of America

WHAT YOU WILL LEARN IN THIS BOOK
How This Book Will Help You and Why

The Paleo Diet is possibly the best way to lose weight naturally and improve your health, it is more than just a diet, it is a lifestyle. You will effortlessly transform your body into the perfect body you were always supposed to have.

Not only that but it has been shown to help people with type 2 diabetes, heart disease, auto-immune diseases, allergies, skin problems and a host of other health issues associated with poor diet. This book will help you understand how to lead a healthy life using the Paleo Diet.

ABOUT THE AUTHOR

Joanne has struggled with weight loss and eating healthy for years. She came across the Paleo Diet through a recommendation from a close friend. Joanne had tried many different variations of diets, the problem is that she could not find the right diet that would help her to beat the overweight and obesity bug that had plagued her for nearly twenty years.

Joanne found the answer and she has made that available to everyone in his book! – All about The Paleo Diet!

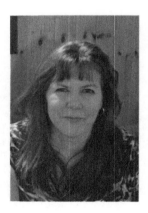

TABLE OF CONTENTS

DEDICATION

I would like to dedicate this book to my family and friends who stood by me the entire time I struggled with my weight gain and rejoiced at my weight loss regime, and to Heather for introducing me to the Paleo Diet. Thanks so much guys!

"Permanent weight loss doesn't come with an on and off switch. It is not something you do for a little while and think it is going to change your body."

- ***Jennifer Hudson***

CHAPTER 1- PALEO THEORY & INTRODUCTION

The Paleo Diet is possibly the best way to lose weight naturally and improve your health, it is more than just a diet, it is a lifestyle. You will effortlessly transform your body into the perfect body you were always supposed to have.

Not only that but it has been shown to help people with type 2 diabetes, heart disease, auto-immune diseases, allergies, skin problems and a host of other health issues associated with poor diet.

Once you realize how amazing you feel and look, you won't go back to your old way of eating, simply because the moment you cheat you will realize how bad those foods make you feel. However don't think you won't enjoy eating anymore, far from it, the paleo diet is not restrictive of calories and you can still eat most of the foods you love!

Understanding the Paleo Theory

The idea behind the Paleo Diet is that we as humans are not eating the foods we are supposed to, the foods we are genetically adapted to eating, the foods we thrived on as caveman, and the foods we became smart eating.

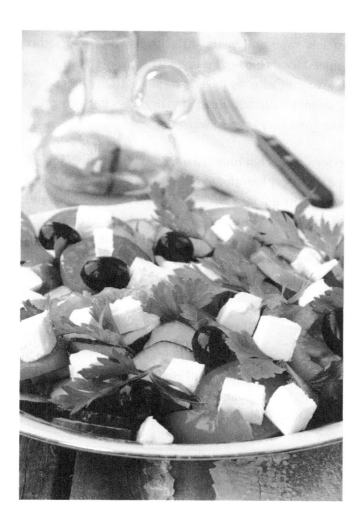

Research shows that during the Paleolithic period, people mostly ate vegetables, fruits, nuts, roots, fish and wild animals. Their diet contained a lot of variety in contrast to today's eating habits which have replaced these wholesome foods with foods high in refined sugars, high fructose corn syrup, breads and cereals (based around cultivated crops like wheat and rice) and pasteurized dairy products.

During the last few thousand years with the dawn of agriculture, we have introduced foods into our diet which we simply would not have been able to cultivate as cavemen. Since then things have gotten worse, we may have advanced in many ways but in terms of our diet we have gone very far backwards.

The typical modern diet is not only full of completely nutrition-less food but most of it is very harmful to our bodies and the evidence is for all to see! Obesity epidemics, diabetes rates soaring, allergies, skin problems (acne), heart disease and cancer. It doesn't have to be this way, these illnesses are preventable (and curable!) through eating like our ancestors ate, the Paleolithic man did not suffer like us and neither should you!

Theory in practice

There are a number of studies which back up the theory. A study by the medical school at the University of Hull in England argues that our Stone Age genes are not adapted to our current lifestyle. Our environment is evolving quicker than we are and as result many chronic diseases and degenerative conditions have developed among western societies.

In a recent study, a team of researchers at the University of California tested this diet on a group of volunteers. They ate the traditional paleo diet and found that their cholesterol levels dropped as well as blood pressure and triglycerides. The researchers found that this diet helped to normalize the body's levels and found that, although not the intent of the study, most of the participants also lost weight.

There have also been observational studies of people isolated from western dietary habits such as a population living on the island of Kitava, Papua New Guinea. Among these people there was a complete absence of heart disease and stroke as well other health problems like acne. Interestingly when these people abandon their traditional dietary habits and adopt western ones their health begins to decline and they too are inflicted with the "diseases of civilization".

Weight Loss with the Paleo Diet

One of the biggest changes in the Paleo diet is taking out carbohydrates. The refined grains in today's diet play a huge role in contributing to excess weight and unhealthy fats in the body. These can lead to diabetes and heart disease over time. The paleo diet removes these unhealthy carbohydrates and fructose, which both contribute to high blood pressure.

Benefits of This Diet

While following the complete paleo diet may be challenging, there are principles of this diet plan that can be followed. Eating unprocessed foods, vegetable-based carbohydrates, and maintaining an active lifestyle are all parts of the paleo diet. The paleo diet has seen great results and it can be extremely beneficial.

Composition of the Paleo diet

As in the case of any food based regimen, to obtain optimum health benefits the paleo diet also allows the eating of certain foods and abstention from some others. The following are the rules that generally are the governing rules of the paleo diet.

* *Emphasis on foods that may fall into the category of what can be hunted or fished.*

* Restricting the eating of processed foods or ones having any preservatives.

* Complete elimination of carbohydrates from grains and legumes.

*Restriction on eating of sugar, salt and dairy products.

* Complete abstention from coffee and reduction in the consumption of alcohol.

*Fruits and vegetables are allowed in unlimited quantities with the exception of potatoes as they are high in starches and in most cases are genetically modified as compared to what was grown in the ancient times.

*While choosing meats, it will be necessary to keep the choice to lean meats, removing excess fat, or it may lead to other medical complications.

* In almost all respects but for the complete abstention from dairy, which happens to be a rich source of calcium, and legumes and grains that are rich in vitamin B6 and B12, the diet more or less abides by the daily nutritional allowance needed by all. The healthy switch for most modern societies to low- processed, low -sodium diet, that has a healthy dose of fruits and vegetables cannot really be derided. Yet it is necessary to follow the diet plan with some prudence.

The low carbohydrates and sodium works wonderfully for those wanting to lower their bad cholesterol levels and also triglycerides levels, but one must be cautious about the manner in which nuts and meats add on to the fat content in the body and how the low sugar levels may to an extent affect the energy levels. No beginner's guide to the paleo diet can quite be complete without a word of caution about the extent to which the diet can succeed in lowering weight. It goes as per every person's metabolic rate and the ability to sustain the diet for a longer period of time.

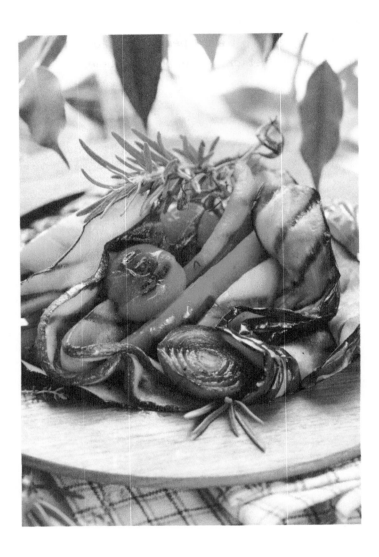

It is necessary to conclude by highlighting the fact that the healthy switch to eating more organic foods does have immense benefits that cannot be ignored in its overall impact on our body irrespective of the diet plan's impact on lowering body weight.

CHAPTER 2- EAT THIS NOT THAT WHILE ON THE DIET

What foods can be eaten?

Quite simply, the foods which are eaten are the foods which we consumed as cavemen. This means eating whole foods, full of nutrients which will help with weight loss and other health issues.

You can eat:

Fruit, Vegetables, Meat, Fish and Seafood, Eggs, Nuts and seeds, Good fats (like olive oil, coconut oil and avocados)

You cannot eat:

Vegetable Oils, Grains (bread, rice, pasta etc.), Starchy tubers (potatoes), Dairy, Sugar

You may be thinking that you will have to give up a lot of foods you enjoy (pizza, cakes etc.). Bear in mind that these foods in their traditional form are not good for you however you can create "Paleo Friendly" versions of most dishes if you crave them.

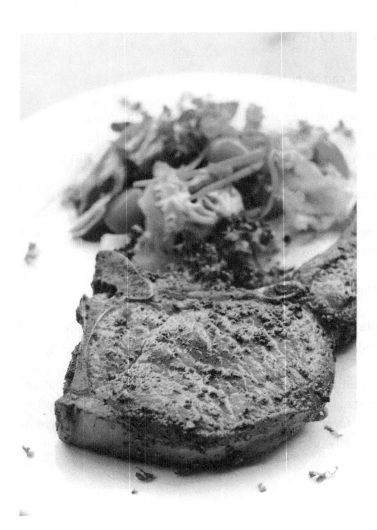

PALEO FOOD LIST

Any foods which cavemen of the Paleolithic era could have consumed are allowed on the paleo diet. These are the foods that mankind is supposed to eat and the foods our bodies are adapted to eating. This way of eating is a logical and consistently successful way to maintain a healthy weight, body and mind.

Use the paleo food list below to get an idea of what foods are allowed on the diet. Note if a food is not on this list then it doesn't necessarily mean it isn't paleo friendly, I have just added some examples. The good thing about the paleo diet is that it is quite easy to think for yourself about whether it is suitable. Just ask yourself, would cavemen have eaten this?

Once you know which foods you can and can't eat you will need to find some recipes to cook. You will however be able to adapt many recipes and meal plans you already use, to a paleo friendly version.

LIST OF FOODS TO EAT ON THE PALEO DIET:

Meat

Beef, Pork, Chicken, Lamb, Turkey, Rabbit, Veal, Goat, Deer, Pheasant, Duck, Goose, Quail and others.

Fish and Seafood

Salmon, Tuna, Cod, Haddock, Sea Bass, Trout, Mackerel, Herring, Anchovy, Swordfish and others.

Shrimp, Crab, Lobster, Prawns, Mussels, Scallops, Clams, Oysters and others.

Eggs

Chicken eggs, Duck eggs, Quail eggs. Ostrich eggs if you are lucky!

Just make sure they are free range.

Vegetables

Avocado, Peppers, Tomatoes, Onions, Broccoli, Cauliflower, Cucumber, Cabbage, Asparagus, Brussels Sprouts, Aubergine, Celery, Carrots, Beetroot, Turnips, Parsnips, Radish, Mushrooms, Butternut Squash, Lettuce, Spinach, Kale, Watercress, Bok Choy and others.

Fruit

Apples, Oranges, Bananas, Kiwi, Grapes, Avocado, Lemon, Lime, Mango, Strawberries, Blueberries, Pears, Peaches, Nectarines, Plums Grapefruit, Pineapple, Pomegranates, Cherries, Apricot, Water Mellon, Tangerine, Coconut, Figs, Dates and others.

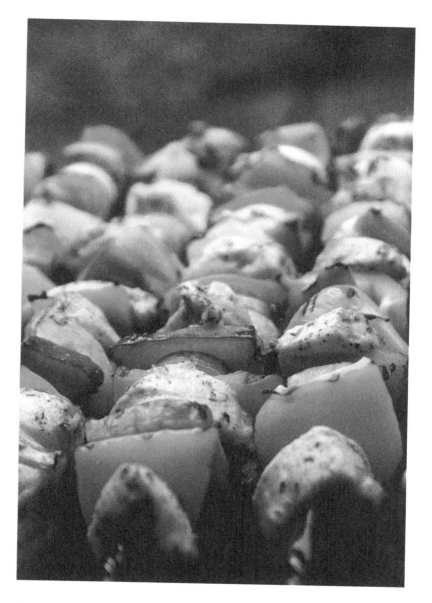

Fats and Oils

Olive Oil, Coconut Oil, Nut Oils, Animal Fat, Avocados, Coconut Milk, Coconut flesh and others.

Nuts and Seeds

Macadamia Nuts, Hazelnuts, Brazil Nuts, Walnuts, Chestnuts, Cashew Nuts, Pistachios, Pecans, Almonds, Sunflower Seeds, Sesame Seeds, Pumpkin Seeds and others.

Herbs and Spices

Coriander, Mint, Parsley, Thyme, Basil, Oregano, Bay Leaves, Sage and others.

Chili Peppers, Garlic, Black Pepper, Star Anise, Cumin, Turmeric, Cayenne Pepper, Paprika, Nutmeg, Vanilla, Cloves and others.

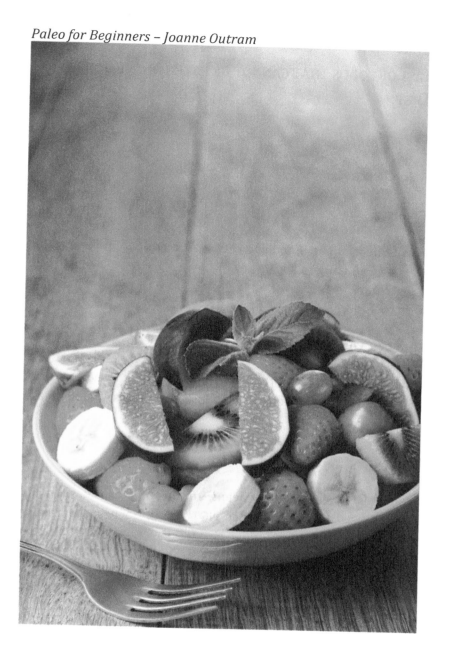

LIST OF FOODS THAT CANNOT BE EATEN ON THE PALEO DIET:

Dairy

Milk, Cheese, Cream, Ice Cream, Yogurt and others

Grains

Rice, Wheat (bread, noodles, cakes, pasta, flour etc.), Barley, Corn, Oats, Rye and others.

Starchy Tubers

Potatoes, Chips, French Fries, Cassava and others.

Note: Sweet Potatoes are OK in moderation as they are full of nutrients. However when trying to lose weight it is a good idea to limit consumption.

Legumes

Beans (black beans, kidney beans, red beans etc.), Peas, Lentils, Peanuts (yes they are legumes NOT nuts!), Soybeans (including soya milk).

Vegetable Oils

Corn Oil, Soybean Oil, Sunflower Oil and other vegetable oils.

Sugar and Sugary Drinks

Sugar, Candy, Soft Drinks, Fruit Juices (they lack the fibre of fruit eaten on its own) and others.

Note: Dark Chocolate with a high cocoa percentage can be consumed (look for 70 per cent cocoa or higher).

CHAPTER 3- PROTEIN POWDER AND WHAT TO DRINK

I'm sure there are many of you out there that like to keep fit, work out and/or do weight training. Of those people, especially the weight trainers I bet you like to increase your protein intake with one of those "delicious" shakes right?

Well if you like to work out regularly then you probably drink a protein shake twice a day. For my friends in this category (I'm not there yet!) it is a very convenient and quick way to add some extra nutrition and protein into their diet whether they are working out that day or not.

The only issue is there are not many paleo protein powders on the market. In fact there are such few choices that many paleo dieters use standard whey protein. Is this a wise choice or is there in fact a healthier more paleo friendly alternative? I will try to answer those questions here.

Is whey protein paleo friendly?

Whey protein is dairy which means it certainly is not paleo. Some people argue it is OK to make this one exception but I mainly disagree. Whey protein contains lactose which causes problems in many people, especially people whose ancestors did not consume dairy. I have tried whey protein myself and did not tolerate it well, this was many years ago though before I had even heard of the paleo diet or cared for nutrition. It may have been a really poor protein powder and I reacted badly to some other ingredient.

Ultimately it is your decision. If you are really into weight training and cannot bear to give up your precious whey protein and seem to tolerate it OK then I won't recommend it but you will still be much healthier overall if this is the only item you "cheat" on. If you do decide to consume whey protein then try and look for a natural one without a huge list of random ingredients.

PALEO PROTEIN POWDER OPTIONS

If like me, you cannot tolerate dairy well or are doing the paleo diet properly (strictly no dairy allowed!) and you still want to gulp down a protein shake to get ripped then there are 2 options; egg white protein and hemp. Sounds tasty right? Well I am a hemp drinker and I actually don't mind the taste, you get used to it and it actually tastes better than anything else I've tried. It only took me a few days to get used to the taste, building up to the required level.

If you are in the UK then you can purchase this protein powder from Amazon for around £12 for Good Hemp Protein Powder Natural 500g. If you are from the USA then there are even more hemp protein powder options on Amazon.

For those of you who really like eggs then you can try the egg white protein powders. I've never gone down that route myself but take into consideration that it is likely to be low quality nutrition made from caged hens which have not been treated well.

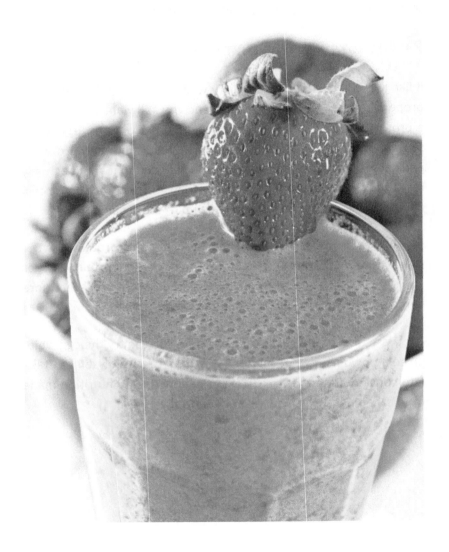

Make your own protein shake

The final option is to make your own paleo "protein" shake, a good friend of mine actually did this for a while and said it tasted really good. The recipe was as follows:

1/2 can of coconut milk

2 tablespoons of almond butter

2 bananas

2 teaspoons cocoa powder

This probably didn't actually contain a huge amount of protein but does contain a massive amount of healthy calories. This is especially useful for people who need to gain weight. For more protein increase the amount of nut butter.

Final Thoughts

Of course the best and only truly paleo option would be just to increase your protein intake through eating more meat and eggs. Drinking your protein and calories cannot be considered natural. But we do live in a modern world, and I still like my breakfast shake, which is made as follows:

200ml almond milk

1 banana

2 teaspoons of coconut oil (optional)

1 scoop of hemp protein powder

½ cup of berries (you can use any, including frozen berries, but I love blueberries for this recipe)

Blend all ingredients and serve.

And to help with pre-menstrual symptoms, then I like to add a teaspoon of cacao powder (or a couple of teaspoons of good quality cocoa powder).

Paleo Alcohol – Does Alcohol fit in with the Paleo Diet?

When it comes to Alcohol most people would probably think there is no room for it on the Paleo diet but this is not the case. There is actually quite a good chance that our Paleolithic ancestors consumed alcohol albeit by accident when eating fruits that had started to ferment. However they almost certainly didn't consume alcohol in the vast quantities many people do nowadays.

I am certainly guilty of overindulging in the booze from time to time. Of course getting plastered every weekend (a pretty normal thing to do here in England!) cannot be great for our health, although there is however evidence to suggest moderate alcohol consumption can actually be part of a healthy lifestyle. This is good news for people who like to drink and are conscious of their weight, health and wellbeing.

Which are the healthiest alcoholic beverages?

Beer

Unfortunately beer is not really Paleo friendly. This is because it is made from grains (normally wheat or barley) and this means it contains gluten. However the amount of gluten found in most beers is small especially Budweiser I am told, which is supposedly almost gluten free.

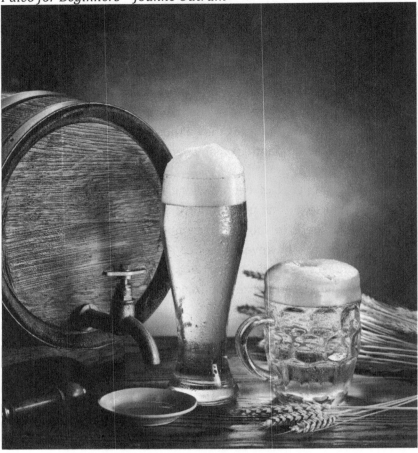

So if the amount of gluten in beer is small then moderate consumption is ok right? Well there is quite a bit of research that suggests even small quantities of gluten can be damaging to a person's health as it damages the gut lining.

Ultimately it probably depends on the person, I cannot give an exact answer and it is a controversial topic in the Paleo world. You will still be improving your health massively if the only gluten in your diet comes from a few beers every now and then rather than massive amounts from bread and baked goods.

Of course you could always have gluten free beer.

Wine

Wine is the closest thing to being fully paleo alcohol. This is because it is made with natural ingredients like grapes in a natural process and is probably at the strength of alcohol we would consume naturally. I'm sure you have also heard of the many studies which claim moderate consumption of wine especially red is good for us as it contains anti-oxidants and resveratrol which may help prevent heart disease (although this is still unclear).

Some people are even massive believers that resveratrol will make you live longer although the quantities in wine are probably nowhere near enough for this effect.

Overall though even if the supposed benefits of drinking wine are still unproven it's certainly not going to damage your health through moderate consumption and it's nice to know there is a chance it may actually improve it. That is a good enough reason for me to continue drinking wine.

Spirits although not natural and certainly not consumed by our Paleolithic ancestors are probably not bad for you in moderation. This is because the distillation process means gluten cannot be present. However this only applies when drunk straight on their own, if mixed with sugary drinks like coca cola or lemonade then you will obviously not be drinking paleo. Good news though for people who like to sip on a glass of whisky every now and then.

Some cocktails can be ok, a mojito mixed with soda water, mint and lime is fine. I'm sure you can use your imagination to create some others.

So moderate alcohol consumption with the right drinks is ok?

That is how I see it and how I will continue, you will have to make your own choice but there is probably not any real health issues caused by occasional moderate drinking especially if you stick to wine and spirits.

Alcohol helps reduce stress, relax in social situations and have a good time which for me fits into the Paleo lifestyle. There are also possible health benefits of wine and even other alcoholic beverages and it may improve insulin sensitivity.

Just remember try not to drink to excess (I know easier said than done!). Not only might you embarrass yourself and have nasty hangover the next day but you may be damaging your overall health.

CHAPTER 4- THE SIMPLE PLAN FOR PALEO SUCCESS

The shops and markets are full of different types of foods, desserts and drinks. With so much food out there, it can be difficult to know what you should stay away from when you are trying to lose weight. What foods fit into your diet well and what foods can cause major setbacks? That is what we are going to help you with right now! There are many sites and articles that tell you what you should be eating, but they forget to mention what you may want to stay away from. Here are some foods that will interfere with you reaching your weight loss goals.

1. Foods that Contain Refined Starch

There are many foods that contain refined starch that you should surely avoid when you are trying to shed a few pounds. This could be white bread, pasta, white rice, potato chips / crisps and French fries. You may be surprised to learn that even muffins aren't that great for you because of refined starch! This refined starch causes these foods to be very high in calories. It makes it even worse when most of these foods are paired together with other items that are high in calories such as butter on your muffins and high calorie sauce on your pasta noodles.

You should do some research and actual searching in the stores to find food items that do not have refined starch. For example, there are many items that taste and look like potato chips minus all of the fat!

2. Baked Foods

Yes, you know what this means! You should steer clear of cookies, Danish pastries, pies, cakes and more. The calories that you will take in when you consume these items are empty, which means that they provide absolutely no nutrients that your body needs. Because they are empty, this means that they aren't as filling and you will want to continue eating more and more of them.

3. Mayonnaise

This is a very bad condiment for your body. Ten grams of mayonnaise has 61 calories, which is a very small amount and a lot of unneeded calories. Say you add an ounce of mayo to your French fries or your sandwich, you will be adding 180 extra calories! Stop and ask yourself, is it really worth it? Not when you are wanting those extra pounds off of your tummy area.

Butter is another food item that is very bad for you. One ounce of butter typically has around 210 calories. This means that when you butter your toast or you melt a bit over your vegetables, you are adding a lot of calories to your diet without even realizing it. Instead of eating butter on your toast, try adding a bit of almond butter!

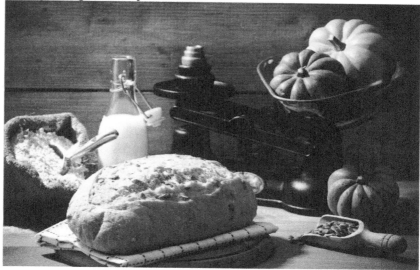

4. Saturated Beverages

It has been shown that the main source of calories American's take in are in sugary drinks and we Brits are just the same. This doesn't just mean fizzy pop, it also means energy and sports drinks as well. These drinks have a lot of calories that you can be using for solid foods instead. Eight ounce of fizzy pop will have about 100 calories if not more, that is 100 calories that can be spent on food that will actually fill you up for a while. Healthy food, of course!

Coffee is another one that you may want to stay away from when dieting as well.

It is best to stick to the water. If you don't enjoy the taste of water, you can always buy fruit juice flavored packets that can be added to a bottle of water. They have very few calories and taste just like regular juice. Or better still; infuse your water with fresh fruits. A jug of water with slices of lemon, cucumber and a few sprigs of fresh mint makes a delicious detox water.

5. Fast Food

You may think that this sounds obvious, of course no fast food when you are dieting and trying to lose weight. However, it is important that you understand just how important it is to stay away from fast food when you are trying to lose weight. Fast food can get in the way of you losing weight much more than you realize. Whether it's burgers, French fries, tacos or pizza, they are all filled with fat and calories that are very unhealthy for your body. They can interfere with your diet so easily because fast food is always available to you and it is so simple to go through a drive through rather than cook a meal at home. If you are going to eat fast food, try eating a salad with light dressing and low-fat yogurt (not strictly paleo but better for you than a typical fast food meal).

CHAPTER 5- THE PRO'S, CON'S AND SUCCEEDING ON PALEO

A Template for Success

This is one of the questions that comes up when someone is beginning the Paleo diet: *will the benefits be sustainable in the long term?* To answer the question, it really depends on a number of factors. I like to consider "the Paleo Diet" as a template. Being a template, we can use it as a framework for our healthy diet lifestyle. Paleo, as per Loren Cordain's book, has however always been a moderate carb / low saturated fat diet.

If an individual is metabolically derange/insulin resistant/overweight then it makes sense to be on a low-carb diet. However, if you do a lot of physical activity for example, then it makes sense to have a paleo diet that has some moderate to high amount of carbohydrates as you will definitely need that fuel.

If there is one thing I have learned from eating paleo, it was never dogmatic.

Of course you can argue that not following a diet 100 per cent is not a good thing because it will be subjective. I don't think subjectivity is a question here but it comes down to the individual. If you can take dairy – then have a little in your diet. I personally can cope with a little milk in the odd cup of coffee.

Experimentation is the key, to find out what suits you. We are all different. The important thing is that going paleo will bring you to the correct path of having a healthy lifestyle.

The paleo diet allows the follower to eat animal proteins through quality lean meats, besides eggs, and fish. In addition, they can eat fruits and the non-starchy varieties of vegetables. Nuts and seeds can be eaten in moderation along with healthy fats such as olive oil and fish oil along with herbs and spices. This is because paleo diet belongs to an era where our ancestors did not suffer from the modern day woes induced by diet. This kind of diet which is rich in fruits and vegetables besides lean protein, omega-3, as well as polyunsaturated fats will make the body use food rather than storing it as fat.

Consumption of legumes and grains can block some key digestive enzymes, besides promoting inflammation and can be the cause of various autoimmune diseases.

There is concern about the paleo diet not being able to provide enough calcium due to non-consumption of dairy. But the fact remains that calcium can be gained by consuming other food stuffs such as leafy greens especially kale and spinach, besides cheese, milk and yogurt. In fact, the acidity of dairy can actually cause calcium to leach from bones in order to regulate the alkaline levels of blood. Thus it is better to opt for these other options for getting calcium as the alkaline nature of vegetables will not lead to the stealing of calcium from your bones.

There can be some real good health benefits by increasing the consumption of fruits, vegetables besides lean meats and healthy fats while cutting the intake of refined sugars, besides bread and other processed fats.

The Cons

Dairy, grains, besides legumes, and starches cannot be consumed. Processed foods and sugars cannot be consumed as well. Alcohol should be limited in quantity, if not eliminated altogether, and restricted to wines and spirits. As per paleo thinking, the human digestive system is not designed to handle refined sugars or starchy carbohydrates, grains, or even legumes or dairy products.

Legumes along with whole grains are known for reducing risk of disease. Besides, they improve insulin sensitivity as well as blood glucose levels. Also, the dietary lectins obtained from legumes as well as grains can boost the good bacteria inside the stomach and aid digestion.

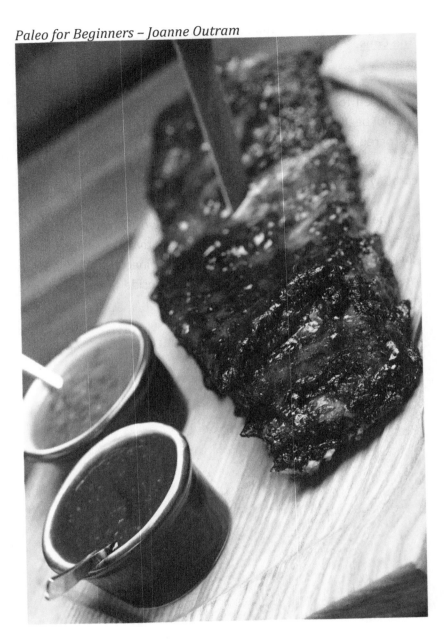

Do note that some varieties of the paleo diet allows for consumption of some of the prohibited food. For example "The Perfect Health" diet which allows eating of safe starches (white rice and potatoes). The paleo diet really is a template that can be adjusted to suit the individual needs.

CHAPTER 6- SLEEP, EXERCISE AND BANNING SUGAR

Some people don't know or simply ignore the importance of sleeping early and getting a good night's rest. A lot of study has been carried our which show the benefits of having adequate sleep.

So what are the major benefits of having a good night's sleep?

1. Helps with Weight Loss

Studies show that if you are going on a weight loss plan, it is very important to have an adequate amount of sleep. It's not just about the type of food to eat, remember to sleep enough as well.

2. Reduce Stress

Controlling stress is very important to our health. It is said to be one of the contributing factor to heart disease. Having enough rest everyday helps reduce stress. For those of us who eat when stressed, this has got to be good news.

3. Improve Metabolism

Lack of sleep reduces your metabolism, which in turn makes you eat more due to the effects of hormones in our body.

4. Increases Energy

Our body isn't a machine. We need ample rest and having good rest will make us feel refreshed and energized the next morning.

5. Boost Immune System

Study suggests that sleeping increases the production of white blood cells. So if you are getting enough rest, the least likely for you to catch common diseases.

Remember to always sleep in the dark. Sleeping in complete darkness helps in the production of melatonin. Melatonin is important in maintaining our body's circadian rhythm so make sure you that once you are in bed, turn off those pesky tablet computers.

Paleo – Stay Away From Sugar

Although sugars are important for proper functioning of the body, excess sugars could be detrimental to our health. Most of the harmful sugars are found in fizzy pop, icings, boiled sweets, chocolate bars and junk foods.

So what are the harmful effects of excessive sugar?

Decreased immunity: Research has shown that people who are subjected to higher doses of sugars have reduced immunity which means that their bodies are unable to fight against infections. Simple sugars such as table sugar, glucose, honey and fructose have the capacity to reduce the effectiveness of white blood cells in engulfing bacteria by up to 50%. However, complex sugars do not affect the effectiveness of white blood cells. It has been observed that if you take 100grams of simple sugars, you reduce the body's ability to fight infection by up to 40%. On the other hand, taking complex sugars does not have any negative implications on body's immunity.

Negative effects on learning, behavior and attention: Various studies have shown that taking too much sugars negatively impacts memory, learning, period of attention as well as behavior. However, the level of this effect is different from one person to the other. This means that different people have different sensitivity levels towards sugars.

Sugar promotes hyperactivity- Various researches have shown that there are people who are more sensitive to sugars than others and also children are likely to be more sensitive to sugars than adults. In a study that tried to compare the sugar sensitivity between children and adults, it was observed that the adrenaline levels in children rose by up to 10 times more than that of adults when both groups were subjected to the same dose of sugars. It is important to note at this point that high adrenaline levels could lead to abnormal behaviors. A child brain is at the stage rapid growth and this explains why the effects of sugar could be exaggerated in terms of learning and behaviour.

Sugar promotes obesity: It has been observed that the more sugar you eat, the more your body will ask for. When you consume sugar, blood sugar levels go up and this triggers the body to release more insulin. The excess insulin will signal the body that you are hungry and therefore you will crave for more food. When there is excess sugar in the blood, the body is stimulated to release Lipoprotein lipase, an enzyme that signals the body to store excess sugar in fat cells. After a short time, this will lead to obesity.

Sugar promotes diabetes: Excess sugars in the blood have been associated with increased cases of diabetes.

Sugar promotes heart diseases: People who take high levels of sugars have high levels of triglycerides in the blood. Triglycerides are bad cholesterol that is stored on the wall of the heart thus hindering proper functioning of the heart.

We should consume food that is rich in fibre. The presence of fibre slows down the rate of digestion which ensures that only a small amount of sugar is released in to the blood stream at a time.

Avoid refined foods such as white bread, white pasta, and white rice and so on. Instead, eat food that is nutritionally dense.

Importance of Exercise to the Paleo Diet

Exercise plays a vital role in improving the overall health of the human body. Advantages of performing regular exercises generally vary from one person to another.

Improving the energy level of the body is a main advantage of doing exercises. Studies say that doing high intensity exercise can burn more calories than lower intensity workouts. Apart from burning more calories, doing high intensity exercise is recommended as the best natural way to improve the functioning of cardiovascular system. Hence high intensity exercise is a perfect choice for all people in search of the best way to improve heart health.

If high intensity exercise is not for you, then just try walking or swimming if you can get to a pool. Some exercise is better than none at all. And, if you are really struggling, then consider finding a personal trainer or getting an exercise buddy.

Proper metabolism plays an important role in improving the health of body. Exercising has been found to be very effective to increase the production of Human Growth Hormone. Studies say that production of HGH or Human Growth Hormone can be increased up to 450 percent after the workout time.

Exercise, really is one of the best and most common natural remedial measures recommended for people suffering from obesity troubles. Apart from improving physical health, exercising has also been found to be very good for mental health.

Reducing stress is another great of exercise, which is probably why you find so many executives and business owners in the gym every day. It increases blood circulation and flushes out toxins from body. If you are in search of the best way to eliminate the accumulation of toxins in body, never hesitate to do some kind of workout.

CHAPTER 7- PALEO SWEET TREATS

One of the things I like to focus on, with my spiritual growth, is the optimum functioning of my body. I have, along my journey, adopted the view that my body is my temple, and I should treat it as such. This means looking after myself. But those of you who know me, will attest to my laziness – I am not really one for going to the gym to keep fit, and I have a sweet tooth.

BUT, even a temple deserves a few sweet treats.

So, when it comes to sweet treats, there are a few paleo "cheats" that allow the indulgence of a sweet tooth. Baking the paleo way, required a few items that were new to my store cupboard: almond flour, coconut flour, coconut oil and coconut milk. All these items can be sourced on Amazon or your local health food store. Both almond flour and coconut flour are a little expensive, but the recipes require a lot less than when using traditional wheat flour.

I have included here some of my favourite breakfast treats, cake, apple pie and ice cream!

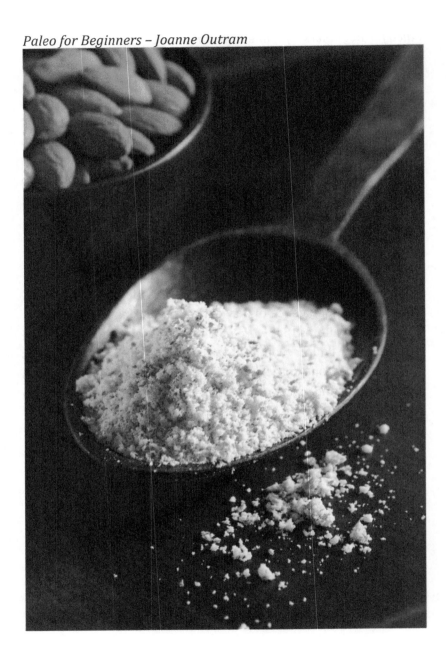

Paleo Dark Chocolate Brownies

2 cups almond flour
1 cup cocoa powder
 1 scoop vanilla protein powder (optional)
1 teaspoon ground cinnamon
1 teaspoon baking soda
Pinch of salt
1 cup melted grass-fed butter (I substitute this with coconut oil)
1/3 cup honey or maple syrup (I use maple syrup)
2 eggs
1 cup coconut milk
2 teaspoons vanilla extract
1 cup dark chocolate chips

Directions

Preheat oven to 325°F / 160°C.

Place the flour, protein powder, cocoa powder, cinnamon, baking soda, and salt in a bowl and combine well. Add the butter (or coconut oil), honey (or maple syrup), eggs, coconut milk, and vanilla and mix until combined. Stir the chocolate chips in last.

Line a brownie tin (I used 8×8inch, can use a larger one if you want thinner brownies) with baking paper or grease the pan. Spoon the brownie mixture into the tin and smooth the surface of the mixture.

Place in the oven for 30-35 minutes.

Makes approximately 16 brownies.

Paleo for Beginners – Joanne Outram
Apple & Cinnamon Breakfast Cake

4 regular size apples, core and chop, but do not peel
½ cup water
1 tablespoon ground cinnamon (plus an additional ½ teaspoon)
1 teaspoon vanilla extract
2 tablespoons coconut oil
9 eggs
2 tablespoons maple syrup / or a sugar free option of 3 dried medjool dates
3 tablespoons of coconut milk
2 tablespoons of coconut flour
¼ teaspoon of baking soda
Pinch of salt

Directions

Preheat oven to 350°F / 180°C.

Sauté the apples, water, vanilla extract, cinnamon & dates (if using) until the mixture looks like apple pie filling. Then add the coconut oil and stir until the oil has melted. Then allow to cool for a few minutes whilst you prepare the rest of the mixture.

In a bowl, whisk the eggs, coconut milk, flour, ½ teaspoon of cinnamon, syrup (if using), baking soda & salt. Combine well, then add the apple mixture.

Line a baking tin (I used 8×8inch) with baking paper or grease the pan with a little coconut oil. Spoon the mixture into the tin.

Place in the oven for 50 minutes or until the top is golden, making sure that it is cooked in the middle. When cold, cut into portions. You can freeze these.

Makes approximately 8 portions.

Individual apple pie

3 tablespoons almond flour
3 teaspoons coconut oil, melted
½ teaspoon vanilla extract
½ large apple or 1 small apple, diced
½ teaspoon almond butter
1 tablespoon coconut butter, melted
Cinnamon, a good pinch should suffice
Pinch of salt

Directions

Preheat oven to 350°F / 180°C.

To make the 'crust', mix together the flour, vanilla extract, cinnamon and salt. Grease a 2x2inch ramekin dish with some of the coconut oil, then press in the mixture.

Combine the apple, remainder of the coconut oil, butters, salt & cinnamon. Then spoon into the ramekin dish.

Bake for 15 minutes.

Apple & spice cookies

1 cup almond butter
½ cup honey
1 egg
1 teaspoon baking soda
½ teaspoon salt
½ apple, diced
1 teaspoon cinnamon
½ teaspoon mixed spice
1 teaspoon grated fresh ginger

Directions

Preheat oven to 350°F / 180°C.

Mix together the butter, honey, egg, baking soda and salt. Then add the diced apple, spices, ginger and stir. Spoon the batter onto a baking tray in round shapes, leaving 1 to 2 inches apart.

Bake for 10 minutes until slightly set. Remove from the oven and allow to cool for 10 minutes before moving onto a cooling rack to finish off cooling.

Makes approximately 9 large cookies.

Luxury vanilla ice cream

1 can coconut milk (28 ounces)
½ vanilla bean (slice lengthwise and scrape out the seeds)
½ cup maple syrup or honey (I use maple syrup)
3 egg yolks
1 teaspoon vanilla essence

Directions

Whisk together all the ingredients (excluding the vanilla essence but including the vanilla bean pod!) in a saucepan. Stir the ingredients continuously over a medium heat, until the mixture coats the back of a spoon, making sure it does not boil. This should take around 8 to 10 minutes.

Transfer the mixture to a bowl and cover with cling film, directly onto the mixture. Place in the fridge and chill for about 2 hours.

Once chilled, take out the vanilla pod and mix in the vanilla extract. Process the mixture in your ice cream maker. There are plenty of non-expensive ice cream makers on the market. I picked up my ice cream maker from Amazon.

When completed, pour the mixture into an air tight container, putting cling film onto the surface of the mixture to avoid freezer burn.

When ready to serve, take out for 30 minutes to soften.

Individual chocolate mug cake

3 tablespoons almond flour
3 tablespoons cocoa powder
2 tablespoons honey
1 teaspoon vanilla extract
1 egg
Pinch of salt
Pinch of cinnamon
1 tsp of coconut oil (optional)

Directions

Mix in a microwave safe mug, then microwave for 2 minutes.

You do not have to include the coconut oil but if not, the cake may be a little dry.

Paleo for Beginners – Joanne Outram

Breakfast Crepes

3 eggs
½ cup coconut milk
2 tablespoons coconut flour
1 tablespoon vanilla extract
Coconut oil to grease the frying pan

Directions

Whisk all ingredients.

Heat an omelet pan on medium heat and melt a small amount of coconut oil. Cook for 1 to 2 minutes until able to scoop the crepe onto a spatula and flip. Cook for a further minute.

Serve with berries and a little maple syrup.

Makes approximately 6 crepes.

Banana pancakes

2 eggs
Banana (can use a ripe banana)
Coconut oil to grease the frying pan

Directions

Mash the banana with a fork and then whisk in the eggs.

Heat an omelet pan on medium heat and melt a small amount of coconut oil. Cook for 2 to 3 minutes until able to scoop the pancake onto a spatula and flip. Cook for a further minute.

Serve with strawberries or blueberries and a little maple syrup.

CPSIA information can be obtained at www.ICGtesting.com
Printed in the USA
BVOW10s0145050115

381904BV00003B/1/P